The Amazing Keto Diet

Benefits, Low-carb, Lower Cholesterol, Fat Burn, Weight Loss, Effective Ketogenic Diet, More You Need to Know

Debra Leo

Disclaimer

The information in this book is for educational purposes only. It should not be taken as a direct advice from medical care personnel. The advice from your physician remains the best source of information. Therefore, always seek medical advice from your doctor to ascertain if your body or health condition allows for keto diet explained in this eBook.

All the information in this book is based on experience and research. It will strive to guide you on everything you need to know about the keto diet as a beginner or an experienced person.

I made sure that you get the best you can find but consultation from your doctor is required before you start. It is your responsibility to evaluate and confirm the information in my ebook with other sources. Get the involvement of your physician or any qualified medical health care professional before you embark on the keto diet journey.

TABLE OF CONTENTS

CHAPTER ONE
Introduction

A growing number of people have come to discover an amazing way to keep the body healthier and stronger. The common idea among people is that you need to eat a lot of carbs and other foods to give the body the energy it needs for fuel. This seemingly bright idea does not work the way we think. The body needs a conscious and intentional type of diet to make and keep it healthy.

Hurray, keto diet comes to the rescue, debunking the age-long idea that carbohydrates are the body's all-sufficient source of fuel. The human body is one simple and complex system that can be guided towards a healthy state. A keto diet or ketogenic diet is the secret to the treatment of certain diseases in children and adults. This is why many experts recommend this healthy diet plan for their patients.

It is not a miracle cure but it could hold the key to a new door of wealth and health. With only a basic understanding of the keto diet, you can transform your body into the level of health you had been dreaming of. Dreams come true, and a keto diet can make that dream real for a very long time.

Keto and Keto Diet

If you are wondering what a keto diet means, you are about reading one of the most informative and helpful books out there. When you hear people talking about or taking a keto diet, it means their daily meals are made up of moderate proteins, low-carbs, and a high amount of fats. This kind of diet is effective in promoting weight loss and the overall health of the body. Keto diet has a history of great performance, which is why many doctors and health professionals highly recommend it. You can lose excess body fat and deal with type 2 diabetes by subjecting yourself to the keto diet for a specific period of time.

The aim behind this amazing diet is to provide more calories from protein and, especially fats, and fewer calories from carbohydrates. That means you have to reduce the number of carbohydrates you take on a daily basis to achieve your health goals. Some of the carbohydrates to or cut down on are white bread, sugar, pastries, and soda. The body requires more than 50 grams of carbohydrates per day to supply the energy its needs. When less than the required amount of grams is supplied, the body quickly runs out of fuel for its usual energy. This makes the body turn to other sources of fuel such as protein and fats. It is this break down of proteins and fats that result in weight loss or reduction in body fat. This process is called ketosis, and is the major aim of a ketogenic diet.

How the Word "Keto" Originated?

The word "keto" was so named because of the effects the diet causes in the body. When a person is on a keto diet, the body produces "ketones", which are little molecules that have the power to supply fuel to the body. These little soldiers act as powerful alternatives to the body's glucose fuel supply. They come in when blood sugar, otherwise known as glucose, is in short supply. For instance, when you consume fewer carbohydrates in your daily meals, your liver will begin to produce ketones from available fat. These ketones that your body produces become the source of fuel to your body system and the brain. You need a lot of energy in your brain every day to function at your best. The brain as an organ easily runs out of energy from glucose but it can live on energy from fats for a longer period.

When you are on a ketonic diet, your body focuses on producing energy by burning fat all day for as long as the fat is available. There are two main sources of energy to the body: **fat** and **glucose**. And since there is a suspension of the latter, the former becomes the major and only source of fuel. Usually, if there is a drop in the insulin of the body, the body increases the amount of fat it burns 24/7. It becomes easier to gain direct access to fat storage and burn them off.

If you want to get rid of body fat or lose weight, this is a simple way to do it.

In following a keto diet, your body continues to receive a steady supply of energy. You never have to worry about the upward and downward shoot of your sugar levels associated with high carbohydrates intake because they will never happen. This can help you stay alert and focused on your daily tasks and the week ahead.

The production of ketones in the body brings about a metabolic state known as ketosis. The fastest way you can put your body in this state is by fasting. When you do not eat anything for some time, the body goes into ketosis. However, you cannot fast forever, so your best option is a keto diet. Keto promotes ketosis, and you can follow this diet for as long as you want.

The keto diet was usually prescribed to people suffering from seizure disorders. This is because ketones and beta-hydroxybutyrate produced by keto diet can help to minimize seizures. When people found out about this useful diet, they started following, which amazingly led to weight loss and other benefits we know concerning keto. When you consume more carbs, the body stores them in the form of fluid to produce energy. But when the body receives no carbs, it loses the fluids. This is what leads to the carbohydrates cravings that people experience. Eating more fat will reduce these cravings and make the stomach feel full.

It makes real sense to be on a diet that helps you lose some fat and enjoy a good body weight. Keto diet has a lot of benefits that you are about to discover in subsequent pages. You don't have to fast for a long time anymore and put your health at risk. With the keto diet, you are on your way to getting most of the benefits of fasting and much more.

CHAPTER TWO

Who Should Not Go on Keto Diet

People have different body systems and sometimes, health conditions can limit the things you can do or the extent you can go. While there are several benefits of keto, the ketogenic diet is not for everyone. You have to be sure your health condition allows you before you do it. If you are in doubt whether or not you are qualified to embark on this amazing journey, see your doctor for advice. Don't give this diet a try without finding out first if it is safe for you.

Let's take a peek at the types of people who should stay away from the keto diet.

Type 1: Women who are Pregnant

Experts strongly advise that pregnant women should avoid going on a keto diet. The duration of pregnancy is not the time to think of losing weight or going the keto way. If you are pregnant, that means another life is forming inside you and you don't want to deny it essential nutrients. When you cut food nutrients, it becomes hard for the baby to have all it needs to grow healthy and strong. During pregnancy, you need vegetables, fruits, and whole grains to promote the healthy development of the baby. You also need folate, choline, and B vitamins to keep your body healthy and strong. Avoid going on a keto diet while pregnant, and if you are worried about gaining weight, ask your doctor to help you put together a nutritious and healthy meal plan. Eating food that lacks all nutritional bases will stall the development of the baby, so doctors do not recommend a keto diet for pregnant women.

Type 2: Women Who Breastfeed Babies

Although research is still ongoing in this area, doctors would advise that breastfeeding women should eat carbs moderately instead of going too low on carbs. In fact, it is suggested that women with babies need more calories than pregnant women. Cutting down intake may affect the supply of breast milk thereby denying the baby of essential food. Breastfeeding mothers need to take adequate water and drink a glass of water each time they nurse their babies. If you are a nursing mother and planning to go on a keto diet, you may need to reconsider your decision. Ketogenic diet leaves out fruits and vegetables which contain water, putting you at risk of dehydration. It is better to avoid it and wait for the time you have weaned the baby and in a good shape before you embark on the keto diet.

Type 3: People with Digestive Disorders

If you have digestive problems, you are going to have a hard time with the keto diet. The reason is that the diet has low carb content, and low carbs mean an insufficient amount of fiber. Fibers help in the digestion of foods, and without it people with irritable bowel syndrome and chronic constipation will have difficulty in going through the process. On average, you need between 25 and 35 grams of fiber each day. Experts are worried that the low fiber content due to low carbs in the keto diet can have a negative effect on people with digestive disorders. So if you are suffering from digestive problems, it is better to avoid low carb meals and, definitely, keto diet should not be on the menu.

Type 4: Children Suffering from Seizures

In the past, the ketogenic diet was used for the treatment of seizures, especially in children. But since they are children, you may not know how they are going to react to it. If a child is suffering from seizures, you have to make sure there is a balance of macronutrients (carbohydrates, protein, and fat) in the body before further action. However, thorough supervision from a medical professional is advised if the child should be placed on a keto diet.

Type 5: People with High Risk of Osteoporosis

When the bone of a person is both brittle and fragile, such a medical condition is called osteoporosis. There is enough evidence to show that a keto diet is not a good fit for people with this disease. A recent experiment conducted on rats and mice showed that feeding animals with the diet recommended in keto will cause bone mineral loss. Findings also show that children placed on a keto diet eventually begin to experience poor bone health. There is no known explanation as to why these things happen. However, taking precautions or avoiding future problem is a good way to stay safe. So people with osteoporosis or poor bones should not follow the keto diet.

Type 6: People with Removed Gallbladder

The function of the gallbladder is to produce bile for the breakdown of dietary fats. If there is no organ that breaks down fat, it is highly risky to eat food with high-fat content. Keto diet is high in fat and a person without gallbladder may find it difficult to go through it. Somehow, the liver also produces bile and is an alternative for the gallbladder.

Personal experiences gathered from people show that some people with removed gallbladder can go through keto diet successfully. However, it is safer to go on a diet that has shorter fatty acids like coconuts. It is also recommended that you discuss it with your doctor before doing anything.

Type 7: People Who Engage in Intensive Activities

We mentioned that fat produces energy in the absence of glucose produced by carbohydrates. There are times when fats do not provide energy for certain activities or people who are into rigorous training. Although this area is still hotly debated, it is possible that activities such as martial arts do not benefit from keto dieting. A sport like running is compatible with keto and is even highly encouraged. Individual body endurance counts because while some may have no problem going on low carb, others may find it difficult to function without their usual carbohydrates intake.

But there is a way to handle the shortage of carbohydrates in the diet. Athletes and people in intensive activities can add a little more carbs in their diet during training days and go on the normal keto diet during off days. This process is known as cyclic keto, meaning upping your carbs by 200 or 230 grams only during training days to enhance the regenerating ability of your cells.

Type 8: People Suffering from Anorexia

Anorexia needs to be mentioned here because of the challenges it poses the person who suffers from it. People with this problem have a nagging fear of weight gain. They are afraid that a little fat can distort their body image and give them what they did not want. This fear intensifies at the thought of eating fat, and the keto diet is all about more fat and fewer carbs and proteins. So to minimize the possibility of gaining weight, anorexic patients tend to avoid dietary fats. The human body cannot function well without dietary fat, which is why it is dangerous to anorexic patients.

The danger is that a person with anorexia may want to omit fats in the keto diet. The strong temptation will always be there since anorexia is a mental disorder. Without the proper amount of fat, the victim is heading towards a danger zone. The absence of fat in a diet means possible starvation and the feeling of not being satisfied even after a meal. But with close medical monitoring, anorexic patients can be encouraged to go through with the diet and experience proper restoration of body and brain.

Type 9: People on Medications

The ketogenic diet can reverse chronic illnesses and mood disorders. But persons on medications will experience side effects in the first few weeks if they go on a keto diet. Some of the risky conditions for the keto diet are a drop in blood pressure, a sudden drop in sugar level. The presence of medication increases the above effects and causes extreme reactions in the body persons. There are many other situations that are highly risky with keto diet but these examples are important to highlight. If you are under any medications, consult your doctor for professional advice and, perhaps, supervision.

CHAPTER THREE
What Keto Diet Looks Like

Keto diet has become popular among older and young adults. The reason is that it is effective in dealing with weight loss, epilepsy, and diabetes. There is an ongoing research on the extent of the effectiveness of this diet on cancer and Alzheimer's disease. When you are on a keto diet, you limit your carbs intake between 20 to 50 grams per day. This is the easiest part since you can measure each food component without any difficulty.

The challenge is when it comes to choosing the right nutritious foods.

Here are some of the healthy foods that should constitute your healthy keto diet.

Vegetables with Low-Carbs

You should go for non-starchy vegetables that have low carb and calorie content but are high in vitamin C and other important minerals. Keep in mind that vegetables contain fiber that does not digest in the body. You may need to first find out their level of digestibility before adding them to the menu. Although most vegetables are low in carbs, eating starchy vegetables such as potatoes, beets or yams could make you go beyond your diet requirement. Other low carb vegetables like cauliflower and broccoli are known to be effective in reducing heart disease and cancer. It is advisable, however, to use low carbs foods when planning a keto diet.

Avocados

Avocados are some of the healthy foods you can find. They contain a high number of minerals and vitamins in addition to potassium, which is a mineral deficient in many people. When there is a high amount of potassium in the body, it becomes easier to maintain keto dieting. Apart from that, avocados can help to improve triglyceride and cholesterol levels.

Poultry and Meat

Poultry and fresh meat do not contain carbs but they have high B vitamins and other essential minerals such as potassium, zinc, and selenium. They are rich sources of high-quality protein which helps in preserving body mass when you are on a low-carb diet. A study has shown that older women who consume fatty meat experience high-density lipoprotein (HDL) cholesterol levels 8% higher than those who were on a high-carb, low-fat diet. One thing you should keep in mind about this is that grass-fed meat is the best form of meat you can find. Animals who feed on grass produce more high-quality meat with a substantial amount of omega-3 fats, antioxidants, and conjugated linoleic acid than meat produced by animals that feed on grains.

Cheese

Two things describe cheese: delicious and nutritious. There are many types of cheese and all of them, fortunately, are high in fats, and this makes them good components of a ketogenic diet. One ounce or 28 grams of cheddar cheese contains 7 grams of protein and 1 gram of carbs. Cheese has high saturated fats but there is no known medical evidence that it can cause heart disease. Some studies even show that eating cheese can help to protect the heart from diseases. Conjugated linoleic acid is also found in cheese and helps in reducing body fat while at the same time improving body composition. Also, going on a diet with cheese can protect the body from losing muscle mass common with aging.

Coconut Oil

Coconut oil has all the properties of an ideal food for a ketogenic diet. It has medium-chain triglycerides or MCTs which go directly into the liver and turn to ketones the body uses for fuel. People with Alzheimer's, problems with the nervous system, and brain disorders are treated with coconut oil by increasing their ketones levels. Coconut oil is also helpful in getting rid of belly fat and obesity in adults. A study found that men who took 2 tablespoons or 30ml of coconut oil daily reduced by 1 inch or 2.5cm from their waistline without being placed on any other diet. Having coconut in a diet is indeed a good way to go the keto way.

Seeds and Nuts

Seeds and nuts are some of the healthy foods you can find, and they are rich in fat and contain low-carbs. Eating seeds and nuts regularly helps to prevent or reduce heart disease, depression, some type of cancer, and other serious diseases. Seeds and nuts have low net fiber content, and they make your stomach feel full and able to absorb fewer calories in total. While there are great health benefits derived from seeds and nuts, they vary in the number of carbs they contain.

Here is a good list of seeds and nuts with the number of carbs they contain to help you make the right decision:

Sesame seeds: 3 grams net carbs and 7 grams overall carbs

Pumpkin seeds: 4 grams net carbs an 5 grams overall carbs

Flaxseeds: 0 grams net carbs and 8 gram overall carbs

Chia seeds: 1 gram net carbs and 12 grams overall carbs

Walnuts: 2 grams net carbs and 4 grams overall carbs

Pistachios: 5 grams net carbs and 8 grams overall carbs

Pecans: 1 gram net carbs and 4 grams overall carbs

Almonds: 3 grams net carbs and 6 grams overall carbs

Brazil nuts: 1 gram net carbs and 3 grams overall carbs

Macadamia nuts: 2 grams net carbs and 4 grams overall carbs

Cashews: 8 grams net carbs and 9 grams overall carbs

Dark Chocolate

If you have tried dark chocolate and cocoa, you will understand how deliciously rich in antioxidant they are. The amount of antioxidants in cocoa is so much that it is named "superfruit". Cocoa promotes much more antioxidants than blueberries. Dark chocolate has flavanols that are effective in reducing the risk of heart disease by keeping the arteries healthy and bringing down blood pressure. Chocolate can be added to a ketogenic diet if the person has nothing against this delicious dark substance. However, it is important that you choose dark chocolate containing a minimum of 70% cocoa solids to get the best benefits. One ounce or 25 grams of unsweetened chocolate contains 3 grams of net carbs, while 70 to 85% of dark chocolate has about 10 grams of net carbs.

Olives

Olives in the solid form have the same health benefits as the oil extracted from the fruits themselves. The main antioxidant found in olives is called oleuropein and it has inflammatory properties that may help prevent cell damage. Some studies have shown that regular consumption of olives can stop bone loss and even reduce blood pressure in people. However, the amount of carbs varies from olive to olive depending on size. Half of the carb content in olives is from fiber, which means they are not easily digestible. One ounce or 28 grams of olives has 1 gram of fiber and 2 grams of overall carbs.

Unsweetened Tea and Coffee

These two are incredibly healthy, contain caffeine, and are carb-free drinks. The caffeine content in tea and coffee helps to increase metabolism and may have an impact on the improvement of physical performance, mood, and alertness. People who have regular coffee and tea drinks have shown evidence of significantly reduced risks of diabetes. Those who have the highest number of coffee and tea drinks have the lowest possible risk of suffering from diabetes. There is nothing wrong with having heavily creamed tea or coffee, but tea lathe and "light" coffee are not good for you. They contain non-fat milk and have a substantial amount of carbs flavorings. It is best to avoid such drinks as much as you can.

Cream and Butter

Cream and butter are good sources of fat which you should be on your keto diet plan. Each serving of cream and butter contains a few traces of carbs. In the past, people believed that cream and butter have a high amount of saturated fat which caused heart disease. But several studies have debunked that suspicion and shown that there is no evidence that links heart disease to saturated fat. In fact, moderate consumption of high-fat dairy products can reduce the risks of stroke and heart attack. Like other dairy products with fat content, cream and butter are rich in linoleic, which is known to enhance fat loss.

Shirataki Noodles

This noodle is an amazing addition to your keto diet at any time. They have less than a gram of carbs and contain 5 grams in each serving due to their large percentage of water content. Shirataki noodles come from a viscous fiber called glucomannan which has the ability to absorb close to 50 times its water weight. This fiber slows down the movement of food along the digestive tract by forming a gel. It results in the reduction of hunger and the decrease of a spike in blood sugar, helping to effective manage diabetes and weight loss. There are many types of shirataki noodles, and some of them are rice, linguine, and fettuccine. You can eat them instead of your regular noodles for all your different recipes.

Berries

A lot of fruits have high-carb content and so are not good for a ketogenic diet. Berries are different and are an exception due to their low-carb and high-fiber content. Some types of berries such as raspberries and blackberries have fiber-content that is equal to that of digestible carbs. They may look tiny but are loaded with enough antioxidants that can reduce inflammation and protect the body from diseases.

To help you make the right choice, here is a list of the carb count of some of the berries you will find:

Raspberries: They have 6 grams net carb content and 12 grams overall carbs

Strawberries: They contain 6 grams net carb content and 8 grams overall carbs

Blueberries: They have 12 grams net carb content and 14 grams overall carbs

Blackberries: They contain 5 grams net carb content and 10 grams overall carbs

Eggs

If you are looking for one of the most versatile and healthiest foods, eggs are good options. A large egg alone has less than 1 gram of carbs and less than 6 grams of protein; a great quality of a good keto diet. Apart from that, eating eggs regularly triggers the hormones that activate the feeling of satisfaction in the stomach. Eggs regulate blood sugar levels, which leads to a reduction in calories for a full day.

When eating an egg, you need to eat the entire egg as most of its nutrients are concentrated in the yolk. Some of the antioxidants in egg yolk are lutein and zeaxanthin, which help in maintaining a healthy eye. Although people often complain that there is a high concentration of cholesterol in egg yolk, this is really nothing to worry about. The cholesterol in eggs does not raise the levels of blood cholesterol in most adults. In fact, egg modifies your LDL (low-density lipoprotein) in a way that helps to prevent heart disease.

CHAPTER FOUR

Keto Diet Breakdown: What to Eat and What Not to Eat

If you are thinking of going on a keto diet, get ready to have a lot of fat, some protein, and a very small amount of carbs in your meal for as long as you want it. That means your fridge, pantries, and shopping list will be filled up with plenty of meat, nuts, fats and oils, seafood, eggs, dairy, and veggies.

To make it easier for you to know what to find, we have compiled a list of what you should eat and not eat on a keto diet.

What to Eat on Keto

Meats

Chicken, ground beef, lamb, bacon, pork, steak, turkey, ham

Fatty Seafood

Tuna, halibut, trout, salmon, catfish, snapper, scallops, cod

Shellfish

Crabs, oysters, lobsters, mussels, clams

Fats and Oils

Butter, eggs, coconut oil, ghee, olive oil, avocado oil, lard, mayonnaise

High Fat Dairy

Hard and soft cheeses, sour cream, cream cheese, heavy cream

Vegetables

Olives, lettuce, spinach, mushroom, onion, cucumber, cauliflower, cabbage, broccoli, zucchini, asparagus, tomatoes, eggplants, pepper, green beans

Berries

Raspberries, blueberries, blackberries

Nuts

Peanuts, almonds, hazelnuts, macadamia nuts, pecans, walnuts and all the unsweetened butter of each nut

Beverages

Champagne, unsweetened coffee, black tea, and dry wine

What Not to Eat on Keto

The list is long and some of the foods on the list may already be your favorite. However, keep in mind what you want to achieve, and try to make the needed sacrifice. This list includes sugars and starches, bread, sweets, corn, potatoes, juice, beer, rice, some fruits, corn, pasta, baked foods, oatmeal, and whole bread.

Let's look at them in detail.

Fruits

Apples, grapes, bananas, mango, melon, watermelon, plums, lemons, limes, grapefruits, pineapple, cherries, peaches

Grains

Sprouted grains, wheat, rye, rice, barley, corn, millet, oats, buckwheat, amaranth, bulgur

Legumes

Pinto beans, kidney beans, black beans, chickpeas, soybeans, lentils, navy beans

Starches

Pizzas, granola, flour, bread, bagels, rice, corn, oatmeal, cereal, pasta, crackers, popcorn, muesli

Low-Fat Dairy

Skim milk, fat-free yogurt, low-fat cream cheese, skim mozzarella

Alcohol

Sweet wines, cider, beer, sweetened alcoholic drinks

Bottled Condiments

Tomato sauce, ketchup, hot sauces with added sugar, BBQ sauce, some salad dressings

Sweet Treats

Pudding, custard, candy, cakes, buns, tarts, pies, some chocolate, cookies, ice cream

Cooking Oils

Sunflower oil, sesame oil, peanut oil, canola oil, soybean oil, grapeseed oil

Sugar and Sweeteners

Corn syrup, cane sugar, saccharin, honey, Splenda, maple syrup, agave nectar, aspartame

CHAPTER FIVE

Amazing Benefits of Keto Diet

Looking at all the long list of what you need to eat and the pain of missing your favorite for a while, what do you stand to gain on a keto diet? Why do you need to go through all the trouble avoiding foods that seem harmless? The answer is keto has the ability to supercharge your body with its low-carb content. If you are having some doubts for a while now, hop in, and let's look at the amazing benefits of a keto diet. It will help you make an informed decision.

Epilepsy

There is enough evidence to show that a keto diet is effective in dealing with epilepsy. Since the 1920s, people who suffered from epilepsy were placed on a low-carb diet, and there were amazing results. Although this was used specifically for children, it is becoming popular among adults in recent years. While on a keto diet, you can take fewer medications or stay without it until the process is over, and there won't have the usual seizures.

Weight Loss

If you want to turn your body into a fat-burning machine, the keto diet is the way to go. It can be beneficial for losing weight and getting rid of that fat you have always wanted to see go away soon. When you are on this low-carb diet, you increase your body's ability of the burn fat, while the fat-storing hormone, insulin, drops significantly. This is the way to lose weight or get rid of fat without going on a fast if you dread the effect fasting may have on your body. Over 30 reliable scientific studies have shown that keto is effective for weight loss.

Control of Appetite

When you are on the keto diet, you are likely going to have control over your previously uncontrollable appetite. This ability helps you feel less hungry and you are not going to keep eating everything and anything in your fridge. That means eating less and having little or no worry about gaining weight or having fat. There is no control better than eating only when you are hungry. If you are on an intermittent fasting, the keto diet can help reverse the struggle with type 2 diabetes. What more? You save money and time by avoiding snacks and other unhealthy foods. From experience, most people eat twice a day by skipping breakfast, and some even take only one meal daily when on a keto diet. Again, having control over your appetite can curb sugar and food addiction problems. Food can be either a friend or an enemy but a keto diet makes food a useful and permanent friend.

Regulate Blood Sugar and Reverse Type 2 Diabetes

It is possible to manage type 2 diabetes with a keto diet, and even reverse the disease in the process. This makes perfect sense since this low-carb diet lowers blood sugar levels, cutting down the need for medication and ultimately reverses the effect of high insulin levels. This goes further to make it possible for a keto diet to keep people from contracting type 2 diabetes in the first place. Yes, if it can reverse it, it can stop it from happening. However, the term "reversing" in this context is making the disease better and improving the control of glucose and the constant need for medications. But it is all about lifestyle changes and keeping it up. If you return to your former unhealthy lifestyle, over time the disease may likely return and advance once again.

Physical Energy and Mental Clarity

Keto energy is not only for weight and fat loss as some people do it to increase physical energy and improve mental performance. During sessions of the keto diet, the brain has no need for dietary carbs any longer. The fuel from ketones and some traces of glucose keeps the brain functioning. There is a steady flow of fuel or ketones moving to the brain during ketosis. This activity prevents the problems of big blood sugar swings, improves mental clarity, concentration, and focus.

Normal Bowel Movement

For those having an irritable bowel movement (IBM), this is good news as they will have no more worries. A keto diet can resolve constant stomach pain, leading to a calm stomach. You will experience fewer cramps, less pain, and improved IBM symptoms. This is definitely the benefit some people are looking for in a diet like a keto. A survey among doctors showed that most of their patients report a dramatic improvement in their IBM symptoms. While this is never expected, it is one of the good "side effects" of the keto diet and a welcomed one. It feels good to have the excessive gas, bloating and pains go away after a long battle using other ineffective methods.

Treatment of Some Cancer

The body is a complex mechanism that stores and burns fat depending on its needs. A hormone called insulin helps in storing and using sugar as fuel to keep the body running. Ketogenic diet burns this fuel quickly so you don't need to keep it stored in the body. The more sugar you burn, the less you need to produce insulin. The lower your insulin production, the less likely you will develop some types of cancer or even the growth of those cancer cells. However, there is an ongoing research to fully establish the effectiveness of this diet on cancer.

Skin Conditions

For a long time, carbohydrates have been blamed for causing skin conditions such as acne. Cutting down on the number of carbs you take a day will certainly help in ridding your face and body of some skin conditions. A ketogenic diet can cause a drop in insulin level, which could prevent the breakout of acne on the face. A study conducted in 2012 indicated that limited carb intake in a keto diet can reduce acne in some people.

Polycystic Ovary Syndrome

Polycystic ovary syndrome can be a serious source of worry in women. This is a situation where a woman's ovaries become larger than normal, forming some fluid-like sacs around the eggs. The cause of this condition has been linked to increased insulin levels, which is one thing a keto diet reverses. A ketogenic diet reduces the amount of insulin the body produces and, along with exercise and weight loss, may help in treating the polycystic syndrome.

Abdominal Cavity Fat Loss

The proportion of fat is not the same in the entire human body. While some parts of the body have a small proportion, others have a large concentration of fat. The location of fat in the body determines the extent of trouble you will have dealing with it. There are two types of fats:

subcutaneous fat and visceral fat. Subcutaneous fat accumulates under the skin, while visceral fat lines around the abdominal cavity, and is common among obese men. Visceral fat is found mostly around the organs, and the excess of this fat is linked with insulin resistance and inflammation. This is what may cause metabolic disorders noticeable in the West today. The keto diet is low in carbs and can help to reduce harmful fat in the body. During a keto dieting, most of the fat loss comes from the areas around the abdominal cavity.

Triglycerides Drop

The fat molecules that circulate in the bloodstream are called triglycerides.

During an overnight fast, the level of triglycerides can cause heart disease. The increase of these fat molecules in sedentary people is linked to carb consumption and especially the notorious simple sugar. Cutting down on the amount of carbs you take will reduce triglycerides in the bloodstream. Also, eating low-fat diet causes triglycerides levels to increase.

Heart Health

When you choose to go on a keto diet, choose healthy foods to get maximum benefits. Healthy fats like avocados are better than less healthy foods. According to a 2017 study that reviewed the impact of a keto diet on humans and animals, there was enough evidence of a drop in cholesterol level, LDL (low-density lipoprotein or bad cholesterol, triglycerides, and an improvement in the amount of HDL (high-density lipoprotein or good cholesterol). If there is a high amount of cholesterol in the body, it can lead to cardiovascular disease or heart problems. The ketogenic diet reduces the effect this cholesterol has on the human body especially the heart. To get the best outcome, always choose healthy foods even among the list of recommended diet.

Wrap Up

While there are several confirmed benefits of a keto diet, it is important that you see a dietician, doctor, or healthcare provider if you want to start a keto diet and have disease or health problems. It is always good to check if you have some underlying conditions such as diabetes, heart disease, or hypoglycemia that pose a potential danger in the safe eating of low-carb foods. Studies are still ongoing in the long term of this diet. You can get amazing results while on keto on the short. It is truly worth it if you are cleared of any medical conditions by your doctor.